Distribution, publication, and copying in any form are prohibited and subject to damages.

TEN HYPNOSES

Copying, publishing, and sharing with third parties are only permitted with the written consent of the author. Please observe the notes on copyright and usage.

Distribution, publication, and copying in any form are prohibited and subject to damages.

Copying, publishing, and sharing with third parties are only permitted with the written consent of the author. Please observe the notes on copyright and usage.

Distribution, publication, and copying in any form are prohibited and subject to damages.

Ingo Michael Simon

TEN HYPNOSES

15

Domestic Violence, Victim Support

Copying, publishing, and sharing with third parties are only permitted with the written consent of the author. Please observe the notes on copyright and usage.

Distribution, publication, and copying in any form are prohibited and subject to damages.

© 2024 Ingo Michael Simon
All rights reserved.
Independently published
www.ingosimon.com

Important Notes for Urgent Attention:
The contents of this book are based on the practical experiences of the author with hypnosis applications and psychotherapy in a trance state. Although the author has strived for the utmost care, errors or misunderstandings in the presentation cannot be completely excluded. Therapeutic work with people and the application of hypnosis are solely the responsibility of the hypnotist. It cannot be ruled out that parts of this book may be misunderstood or that the application of a presented procedure may cause an undesirable reaction in the client. The author also assumes no co-responsibility if work with a client is carried out with reference to the statements in this book.

The Author:
Ingo Michael Simon studied psychology and education and is a hypnotherapist with practices in southwestern Germany and Switzerland. With the help of hypnosis-supported psychotherapy, he primarily treats people with persistent psychological conditions. His practice focuses on anxiety disorders, pathological compulsions, and psychosomatic illnesses. His therapeutic offerings mainly include classical and modern hypnosis applications and the dreamland therapy he developed himself.

Copying, publishing, and sharing with third parties are only permitted with the written consent of the author. Please observe the notes on copyright and usage.

Notes on Copyright and Usage

Copying, publishing, and sharing with third parties is prohibited and only permitted with the written consent of the author. Please observe the following copyright and usage guidelines.

This work has been carefully crafted and created to the best of the author's knowledge and personal experience. It comprises text templates and application guidelines for professional hypnosis sessions. The author is a licensed psychotherapist with extensive experience in psychotherapy, coaching, and personal training using hypnotic techniques and methods. Nevertheless, the author and the publisher assume no liability for the accuracy of information, instructions, and advice, nor for any typographical errors. The author and publisher accept no responsibility or liability for the application of these texts and recommendations with clients or patients, nor for any potential consequences or unexpected reactions. It is expressly noted that the application of therapeutic and advisory techniques and formulations lies solely and entirely within the responsibility of the practitioner. This also applies to adherence to the boundaries of legally regulated medical and therapeutic practices. The fact that a book containing action proposals is freely available for sale does not imply that its application with clients or patients is permitted for everyone.

Distribution, publication, and copying in any form are prohibited and subject to damages.

Copying, publishing, and sharing with third parties are only permitted with the written consent of the author. Please observe the notes on copyright and usage.

Distribution, publication, and copying in any form are prohibited and subject to damages.

Table of Contents

Introduction 9

#1 11

#2 16

#3 21

#4 27

#5 32

#6 37

#7 41

#8 45

#9 50

#10 55

Overview of All Titles in the Series "Ten Hypnoses" 60

Copying, publishing, and sharing with third parties are only permitted with the written consent of the author. Please observe the notes on copyright and usage.

Distribution, publication, and copying in any form are prohibited and subject to damages.

Copying, publishing, and sharing with third parties are only permitted with the written consent of the author. Please observe the notes on copyright and usage.

Introduction

The series "Ten Hypnoses" is very well known in Germany, Austria, and Switzerland as a collection of texts for therapeutic work and is used by numerous psychotherapeutic practices, doctors, therapists, coaches, and other helping professionals. I am pleased to now be able to offer these texts in other countries as well.

Most therapists have their own methods for inducing and deepening trance as well as for exiting trance. Therefore, I have focused on the main part of the hypnosis. The texts in this book can be integrated as the main part into any hypnosis process.

The texts in this collection use various hypnosis techniques. I will not explain these in detail, as I assume that users have the appropriate training. It is also not necessary to understand the exact structure or functioning of the different parts. The texts can simply be read aloud, and they will have their effect.

Decide for yourself which text best suits your client or patient at any given time. You can also combine passages from different texts. It is not about using all ten hypnoses in sequence. It is a selection of possibilities.

I want to emphasize that books cannot replace therapy. Psychotherapy or other therapeutic treatments involve much more. A careful diagnosis is the necessary basis for deciding on the use of methods, including whether hypnosis or one of my texts should be used. Even in this case, preparatory discussions, follow-up discussions during the session, and of course, a therapeutic concept for the sequence of sessions and the content approaches are essential parts of therapy. This cannot and should not be achieved with a collection of texts.

In any case, I wish you much success in your work and I am pleased if my text templates can contribute in a small way.

Ingo Michael Simon

#1

Goal Formulation and Strengthening Willpower

… … You can finally leave behind the time of violence and fear … … because you have freed yourself and are ready to take new paths … …

… … You can finally leave behind the time of violence and fear … … because you have processed past events and now want to be free again … …

… … You can finally leave behind the time of violence and fear … … because you are internally prepared to look forward now … …

… … You can finally leave behind the time of violence and fear … … because with this trance you can embrace new thoughts and new courage … …

… … A new chapter begins … … Freedom begins … …

Mental Alignment

… … You know that you are now safe again and can remain so … … and therefore, you can focus on your own goals … …

… … You know that you are now safe again and can remain so … … and therefore, you find your new path through life … …

… … You know that you are now safe again and can remain so … … and therefore, you start your new life self-determined and strong … …

… … You know that you are now safe again and can remain so … … and therefore, you look forward to taking new paths, new and self-determined paths … …

… … A new chapter begins … … Freedom begins … …

Somatic Alignment (Body Suggestion)

… … Your body now feels truly healing calm and relaxation … … and therefore, you also feel that the inner wounds are healing more and more … …

… … Your body now feels truly healing calm and relaxation … … and therefore, the old fear gradually fades away … …

… … Your body now feels truly healing calm and relaxation … … and therefore, you find strength within yourself to start anew … …

… … Your body now feels truly healing calm and relaxation … … and therefore, you now start your new life self-determined and confidently … …

… … A new chapter begins … … Freedom begins … …

Emotional Alignment (Feeling Suggestion)

… … Deep inside, you let go of fear and find trust in yourself and in life again … … and this life is truly worth it for you… …

… … Deep inside, you let go of fear and find trust in yourself and in life again … … and this life is now determined only by you… …

… … Deep inside, you let go of fear and find trust in yourself and in life again … … and this life unfolds in freedom and dignity … …

… … Deep inside, you let go of fear and find trust in yourself and in life again … … and this life belongs only to you alone ... ... A new chapter begins ... ... Freedom begins ... ...

Behavioral Alignment

... ... You determine what is allowed in your life and only you decide ... ... because by doing so, you free yourself from old and long-overcome connections ... ...

... ... You determine what is allowed in your life and only you decide ... ... because by doing so, you overcome the fear of the past and come to rest ... ...

... ... You determine what is allowed in your life and only you decide ... ... because by doing so, you recognize that life is open to you again ... ...

... ... You determine what is allowed in your life and only you decide ... ... because by doing so, you stand on your own strong ground ... ...

... ... A new chapter begins ... ... Freedom begins ... ...

Consolidation

... ... You stand on your own ground, in the center of your life ... ... and on your strong and self-determined place you remain ... ...

… … You stand on your own ground, in the center of your life … … and again and again you find your sovereignty and strength and assert yourself … …

… … You stand on your own ground, in the center of your life … … because that is where you belong … … that is where you truly belong … … in the center of your life … …

… … Fear fades … … The past is over … … You start anew … … You are the most important person in your life … … You are the most important person in your life … …

#2

Introduction of the Special

… … You have freed yourself from a difficult time and want to live strong and self-determined again … … You want to be strong and confident again, to shape your life confidently and independently … … free from violence …. … completely free … … You know it wasn't always easy to go your own way and determine what was allowed and what wasn't … … But … … you have untangled yourself from these old ties … … Maybe we could already say … … You have completely freed yourself and made a decision … … or it's not quite finished yet and … … You move forward … … with the goal of achieving even more … … You decide for yourself what you want to do … … and what should be … … also what should be achieved in hypnosis … … Maybe you think … … This hypnosis is an important step of liberation … … because you are convinced or think it possible that … … this hypnosis helps to decide self-determined … … or you wait a little longer … … You decide best … … yourself, how the effect of the hypnosis is, because … … You experience it every day ... ... as soon as you are awake again ... ... Maybe you can soon confirm ... ... These suggestions are helpful ... ... or you come to a different result ... ...

Letting Go of the Disturbing/Neutralization

... ... In the past, your life was often marked by fear ... ... Imagine for a moment ... ... You are completely free from fear ... ... Maybe it has actually been a long time or was only rarely so, but you can imagine it ... ... and if it were so, you could say ... ... You are strong and can protect yourself ... ... because you are no longer afraid and strong ... ...

... ... In this liberation, you could then also simply claim ... ... You have complete control over your life ... ... because it would be perfectly clear to you ... ... You decide best yourself ... ... and ... ... No one can stop you ... ... That would be possible ... ...

... ... And maybe it is already possible or partially possible and soon you will realize ... ... Yes, you are truly free from fear ... ... Then much will be easier because freed from the old fear, you stand at a point where you can say ... ... Now your life belongs to you again ... ... But you have time ... ... You are freer and you have already overcome the captivity

… … Violence is over … … A new life begins and … … you decide for yourself … … what happens when … …

Building the New

… … You surely know sayings and idioms … … for example … … Deep inside you lies a very special power … … or … … Deep inside, there is no fear and no uncertainty … … Maybe they are right and … … deep inside, there is always strength and self-determination … …

… … Maybe there was even a time when you lived or decided strongly and self-determined … … Possibly there was a time when it was clear … … You definitely decide for yourself about your life … … because it was also clear … … You are strong enough to defend yourself … … At that time, it was perhaps certain … … You are the most important person in your life … … and today you remember that … … or it's about creating this standpoint for the first time … …

… … Everything has a beginning and it is never too late to take a strong stand … … if it goes easily, then you think … … That really goes quickly … … if it is more difficult, you rather think … … It should go faster …. … because you long for self-determination … …

… … But here and today you don't need to do anything … … In trance, much happens unnoticed and quietly and suddenly we see … … Everything is resolved as if by itself … … We are amazed and recognize … … It works … …

Stabilization and Success of the New

… … You have heard clear suggestions in the words you heard, but maybe you just let them be and did not recognize how they work … … maybe you thought … … The suggestions heard should work optimally … … and how they work … … doesn't matter to you … …

… … You are right … … because in trance you don't need to do anything … … You just need to allow them … … and that is easy … … You have relaxed and found the way into trance … … maybe enjoying the peace and relaxation of your body … … That is what matters … … You don't need to do more … … just relax … …

… … As soon as you can recognize the effect of the suggestions in your waking everyday life, you know … … Now you are truly free … … and … … Now you alone decide … … because then the effect has already fully unfolded and … … your goal is achieved … … That could be as soon as tomorrow or the day after ... ... or a little clearer every coming day of your life ... ...

... ... And if you have experienced this success yourself, you will surely also encourage others who are on a similar path and tell them ... ... You too will experience liberation and freedom ... ... because ... ... Clear suggestions work best ... ... Maybe you will also tell these people ... ... You decide best yourself ... ... because you know that your decision for trance was the right way and you also want to invite others to go their right way ... ... so that they too can say ... ... Everyone decides for themselves about their life ... ... just like you ... ... exactly like you ... ...

#3

Introduction of the Special

You are here because you want to position yourself strong and confident in your new life ... ... That is your goal ... ... You want to be free and without fear ... ... You want to take your life into your own hands and shape it self-determined ... ... So take the following suggestions and you will recognize for yourself which ones you can agree with the most ... ... Clear suggestions, which somehow sound familiar and therefore very good, usually work the strongest ... [hidden reminder of the previous session with hidden instructions] ... These are the really best suggestions ... ... [hidden instruction for the following suggestions] ... ...

... You have ... untangled yourself from old ties ... [5-10 seconds pause] ...

... You have ... completely freed yourself ... and you move forward ... [5-10 seconds pause] ...

... You decide for yourself what you want ... to do ... [5-10 seconds pause] ...

... This is an important step of ... liberation ... [5-10 seconds pause] ...

... You decide best ... you experience it ... every day ... [Now please about 30 seconds pause] ...

... You have ... untangled yourself from old ties ... [5-10 seconds pause] ...

... You have ... completely freed yourself ... and you move forward ... [5-10 seconds pause] ...

... You decide for yourself what you want ... to do ... [5-10 seconds pause] ...

... This is an important step of ... liberation ... [5-10 seconds pause] ...

... You decide best ... you experience it ... every day ... [Now please about 30 seconds pause] ...

Letting Go of the Disturbing/Neutralization

... You are completely free ... from fear ... [5-10 seconds pause] ...

... You are strong ... and can protect yourself ... [5-10 seconds pause] ...

... You have ... complete control ... over your life ... [5-10 seconds pause] ...

... You decide best ... yourself ... [5-10 seconds pause] ...

... No one ... can stop you ... [5-10 seconds pause] ...

... Now ... your life ... belongs to you again ... [Now please about 30 seconds pause] ...

... You are completely free ... from fear ... [5-10 seconds pause] ...

... You are strong ... and can protect yourself ... [5-10 seconds pause] ...

... You have ... complete control ... over your life ... [5-10 seconds pause] ...

... You decide best ... yourself ... [5-10 seconds pause] ...

... No one ... can stop you ... [5-10 seconds pause] ...

... Now ... your life ... belongs to you again ... [Now please about 30 seconds pause] ...

Building the New

... Deep inside there is ... no fear ... and no uncertainty ... [5-10 seconds pause] ...

... Deep inside there is ... always strength ... and self-determination ... [5-10 seconds pause] ...

... You are strong enough to ... defend ... yourself ... [5-10 seconds pause] ...

... You are the most important person ... in your life ... [5-10 seconds pause] ...

... It goes ... really quickly ... and it should ... go faster ... [5-10 seconds pause] ...

... Everything is ... resolved as if by itself, it ... works ... [Now please about 30 seconds pause] ...

... Deep inside there is ... no fear ... and no uncertainty ... [5-10 seconds pause] ...

... Deep inside there is ... always strength ... and self-determination ... [5-10 seconds pause] ...

... You are strong enough to ... defend ... yourself ... [5-10 seconds pause] ...

... You are the most important person ... in your life ... [5-10 seconds pause] ...

... It goes ... really quickly ... and it should ... go faster ... [5-10 seconds pause] ...

... Everything is ... resolved as if by itself, it ... works ... [Now please about 30 seconds pause] ...

Stabilization and Success of the New

... The suggestions heard ... work optimally ... [5-10 seconds pause] ...

... You only need to ... allow them ... that is what matters ... [5-10 seconds pause] ...

... Now ... you are truly free ... Now ... only you decide ... [5-10 seconds pause] ...

... Your goal is ... achieved ... [5-10 seconds pause] ...

... You too experience liberation and ... freedom ... [5-10 seconds pause] ...

... You decide best ... yourself ... [Now please about 30 seconds pause] ...

... The suggestions heard ... work optimally ... [5-10 seconds pause] ...

... You only need to ... allow them ... that is what matters ... [5-10 seconds pause] ...

... Now ... you are truly free ... Now ... only you decide ... [5-10 seconds pause] ...

... Your goal is ... achieved ... [5-10 seconds pause] ...

... You too experience liberation and ... freedom ... [5-10 seconds pause] ...

... You decide best ... yourself ... [Now please about 30 seconds pause] ...

#4

Goal Formulation and Strengthening Willpower

… … Today you find a new and strong standpoint for yourself … … because this way you can most quickly establish inner boundaries that you can also enforce externally … …

… … You are determined to hear and let all suggestions take effect … … because this way you can most quickly establish inner boundaries that you can also enforce externally … …

… … You are ready to take in helpful words into your deep inner self … … because this way you can most quickly establish inner boundaries that you can also enforce externally … …

… … Today you embark on a new path of helpful hypnosis … … because this way you can most quickly establish inner boundaries that you can also enforce externally … …

Mental Alignment

… … You know that freedom begins with a free thought in your head … … and with this thought, you succeed in drawing visible boundaries again and again … …

… … You know that you can only protect yourself permanently with a clear inner standpoint … … and with this thought, you succeed in drawing visible boundaries again and again … …

… … You know that only you have the right to determine your life … … and with this thought, you succeed in drawing visible boundaries again and again … …

… … You know that your life belongs to you, only to you … … and with this thought, you succeed in drawing visible boundaries again and again … …

… … You determine your life yourself … … only you … …

Somatic Alignment (Body Suggestion)

… … The outer posture of the body reflects the inner attitude … … and therefore, you also succeed in radiating strength and self-confidence … …

… … Your body can immediately adopt a strong and confident posture and does so … … and therefore, you also succeed in radiating strength and self-confidence … …

… … Your body already adopts a truly stable and strong posture … … and therefore, you also succeed in radiating strength and self-confidence … …

… … Your body adopts this stable posture in your everyday life, every day … … and therefore, you also succeed in radiating strength and self-confidence … …

… … You determine your life yourself … … only you … …

Emotional Alignment

… … You trust your instinct that warns you of dangers … … and therefore, you protect yourself from attacks by seeking and accepting help … …

… … You owe nothing to anyone else, only to yourself … … and therefore, you protect yourself from attacks by seeking and accepting help … …

… … You deserve to live free from fear and violence … … and therefore, you protect yourself from attacks by seeking and accepting help … …

...... You find courage and trust deep within yourself ...... and therefore, you protect yourself from attacks by seeking and accepting help ......

...... You determine your life yourself ...... only you ......

Behavioral Alignment

...... You overcome your fear and find strength and courage within yourself ...... You say no to everything that burdens your life and go your own way ......

...... You are firmly determined to decide for yourself what is allowed in your life ...... You say no to everything that burdens your life and go your own way ......

...... You go your way with trust and courage and take care of yourself and your safety ...... You say no to everything that burdens your life and go your own way ......

...... You know that every perpetrator is responsible for themselves, and you leave this responsibility with them ...... You say no to everything that burdens your life and go your own way ......

...... You determine your life yourself ...... only you ......

Consolidation

… … The words heard penetrate deeper and deeper … … and therefore, you overcome fear and pity for the perpetrator and continue on your own path … …

… … You recognize more clearly each day that everyone is responsible for their own actions … … and therefore, you overcome fear and pity for the perpetrator and continue on your own path … … As soon as you are fully awake again, you recognize even more strongly that you want to shape your life self-determined … … and therefore, you overcome fear and pity for the perpetrator and continue on your own path … … You alone determine your life … … You free yourself from everything that hurts and oppresses you … … You free yourself and you stay free … … You are and remain free … …

#5

Preparation and Strengthening Willpower

... ... You are ready to take another step into freedom and self-determination ... ... You want to leave the past behind ... ... You want to leave the time of imprisonment and violence behind forever and never allow it again ... ... You have decided to be free and to stay

free ... ... that is why you are here today ... ... that is why you can also follow inner images ... ... and you know that imaginations can lead to convictions and then to truths ... ... That is what you can really use ... ... the truth of a new free life ... ... a free life that becomes more fulfilling and beautiful every day ... ... For this, you don't have to do anything special ... ... Just be here and allow my words to become inner images ... ... Just let all the words you hear become thoughts and images within you ... ... It's very simple ... ...

Letting Go of the Disturbing/Neutralization

... ... You have experienced a (long) time of violence and you have freed yourself from it ... ... You were like a prisoner, could not escape properly until you finally found the strength to say no and end the imprisonment ... ... Now you are starting anew and for that, it is helpful to completely let go of the old chains ... ... Whatever could hold you, now you are free and you remain free ... ... Imagine the chains of the past were like soap bubbles of your memory ... ... You can look at them and understand them and at the same time, you can let them burst and free yourself ... ... There are three such soap bubbles ... ... First, there is the soap bubble of fear ... ... Fear often accompanied you, you did not know how to defend yourself ... ... But today it is different ... ... today you know that fear could hold you ... ... You have freed yourself, you left ... ... You decided not to let yourself be oppressed anymore ... ... You are firmly determined never to let yourself be beaten again ... ... For that, you needed courage ... ... You have this courage, because only in this way could you really put an end to it and leave ... ... Look into the soap bubble of fear and remember ... ... and then let the soap bubble of fear burst ... ... Imagine that you burst it with your fingers, just like that ... ... You don't need it anymore ... ... It should go away forever ... ... It should be past and remain past ... ... You are free ... ... finally free ... ...

Then there is the soap bubble of guilt … … Often you felt guilty, believed it was your fault … … or you thought you had provoked the aggression and violence … … But today you know that this is not true … … It has never been true … … Only the one who hits is guilty … … Everyone is responsible for their own actions … … You were beaten, that was the action of someone else … … You were always innocent and today it is clear to you … … Today you know that and therefore today you can also let the soap bubble of guilt burst … … You don't need it anymore … … Let it burst before your inner eye … … Now … … Then there is still the soap bubble of pity … … Sometimes you thought you had to protect the perpetrator, you stood in front of him and hoped that it would get better someday … … You felt responsible, but today you know better … … Today you know that the perpetrator was and is solely responsible … … You have freed yourself … … You have ended the pity … … Today you transform pity into compassion and recognize that above all you yourself deserve your compassion … … You feel with yourself and thus you become your own friend … … Look at the soap bubble of pity before your inner eye and let it burst … … very consciously and deliberately, let the soap bubble of pity burst because now your time has come ... ... Now you finally have compassion for yourself ... ... Now you finally stand up for yourself ... ... Now you finally protect yourself ... ... with your courage and with your strength ... ...

Building the New

... ... Deep inside you there is a soap bubble of courage and self-confidence ... ... Courage and self-confidence helped you in your liberation ... ... Courage and self-confidence help you to continue to protect yourself ... ... Courage and self-confidence help you to live self-determined and never be imprisoned again ... ... never be imprisoned again ... ... free forever ... ... really free forever ... ... This soap bubble is as stable as a glass ball ... ... You can hold it firmly inside you and recognize that courage and self-confidence are in a truly stable glass ball ... ... and this ball becomes bigger and more stable ... ... Courage and self-confidence are now available to you every day ... ... Now your new life begins ... ... Now your time begins ... ... free forever ... ... free forever ... ...

Stabilization and Success of the New

... ... New courage and new trust accompany you from now on every day ... ... especially when you should feel fear or pity once again ... ... You recognize very well in your waking everyday life that you have become stronger and can and want to stay on your path of freedom ... ... Deep inside you lies the strength that guides and protects you ... ... and with each new day, you recognize more clearly that you are the most important person in your life ... ... that you are worth living self-determined and free ... ... Fear, guilt, and pity burst daily like soap bubbles in the wind ... ... and you remain free ... ... strong and free ... ...

#6

Preparation

… … You want to overcome and let go of old guilt feelings today … … Guilt feelings that were never your own true feelings … … You were beaten and hurt, physically and emotionally … … You have freed yourself from it and therefore it is now time to free yourself from the guilt feelings … … You sought and found help, you allowed help … … So you find help again today … … with an instance you can believe in or in which you can invest hope and trust … … Maybe you want to find help with a guardian angel or with Jesus … … with an inner friend or with your subconscious … … or with yourself … … Whoever hears you, your inner self also hears you … … So you might say … …

Neutralization

… … Dear self in the mirror / Dear God / Dear Guardian Angel / Dear Subconscious … … I know that I am innocent because I have recognized and understood that perpetrators are always responsible for their actions … … I was beaten and hurt, physically hurt and also hurt in my dignity … … I have felt guilty or at least partially guilty for so long, thinking it was also my fault … … But I know better … … My mind knows that this is not true, but I want to internalize it more deeply in my feelings … … Please help me to truly feel innocent and free deep in my feelings … … With your help, I can and will succeed, I know that … … It is my firm will and conviction that I can live free and self-determined again, completely without guilt feelings … … Dear self in the mirror / Dear God / Dear Guardian Angel / Dear Subconscious … … Help me let go of the old guilt that was never my own … … Mind and feeling should go hand in hand … … innocent and free … …

Reorientation

… … Dear self in the mirror / Dear God / Dear Guardian Angel / Dear Subconscious … … I know that I am the one who must take my life into my own hands because I am responsible for the constructive design of my life … … I can and want to gladly bear this responsibility and with your support, I succeed even faster … … I am ready to open myself again to the opportunities and possibilities of life and to look forward … … I know that at the same time I can continue to process the past and understand more and more what actually happened to me ... ... Dear self in the mirror / Dear God / Dear Guardian Angel / Dear Subconscious ... ... Please show me how it works that I can process the past and at the same time look forward and move forward with a cheerful heart ... ...

Attention, Perception, and Self-Acceptance

... ... Dear self in the mirror / Dear God / Dear Guardian Angel / Dear Subconscious ... ... I know that I must accept myself as I am ... ... how I feel and think ... ... I want to accept myself, with all my strengths and all my weaknesses because I increasingly recognize that both sides are special ... ... What I have considered guilty weaknesses are actually just my traits and characteristics ... ... and I want to try to live with all my traits and make the best of myself and my possibilities ... ... in a life without guilt feelings ... ... in a free life ... ... I know I can do that with your support ... ...

Outlook and Self-Care

... ... Dear self in the mirror / Dear God / Dear Guardian Angel / Dear Subconscious ... ... Please also help me to deal with myself considerately ... ... especially when I blame myself or feel occasional guilt feelings, although my mind knows that I am innocent ... ... Then I want to be patient with myself and trust that I can let go of these guilt feelings very soon ... ... For your support in this, I thank you and also myself, because I know that part of your help is always my self-help ... ... Help from my deepest inner self for me ... ...

Consolidation

... ... Now you can rest a little more because you have taken another very important step ... ... You have asked a trustworthy instance for help and thus also an inner instance in you ... ... So you can trust in double help ... ... So your deepest inner self adjusts to doing everything that helps you overcome and let go of old guilt feelings ... ... So you experience new liberation with each new day ... ... So you can shape your new life every day and be free ... ... truly free ... ... You are and remain free ... ...

Preparation

... ... Today you want to find trust within yourself again ... ... You want to be free and stay free ... ... You want to draw and signal clear boundaries outward to protect yourself ... ... That is important ... ... At the same time, you want to find self-confidence and also trust in other people to participate openly and constructively in life again ... ... All these feelings are within you ... ... Self-confidence exists deep inside you ... ... Hope and trust exist deep inside you ... ... So you find the way to your deep feelings and thus the way to your potential and to new trust ... ... Trust in yourself ... ... in your feelings, in your instincts ... ... Your subconscious helps you with this because it hears and understands every word I say ... ... And every word you can agree with becomes your own word ... ... Then it is as if you were saying all these words yourself or speaking them inwardly ... ... So you are also the one who says ... ...

Self-Encounter and Self-Care

… … I turn my gaze inward, feel into myself to recognize my true feelings and find trust in life and in my fellow human beings again … … and my subconscious opens its doors and lets me actually better recognize my feelings … …

… … I want to find hope and trust again in the depth of my feelings and at the same time feel safe because I can rely on my feelings … … and gently and trustingly my inner self meets me and invites me to look deeper and deeper … …

… … With interest and openness, I find myself in the depth of my emotions and moods and discover caution, trust, and hope there … … and my subconscious, this careful and protective part of me, comes to meet me openly and kindly … …

Self-Acceptance and External Impact

… … I am ready again to encounter my feelings and thus also my fear and caution to find trust in myself and my instincts again … … and my fellow human beings meet me trustingly and kindly on my way … …

… … I accept my need for protection and my caution and step out again step by step … … and thus my fellow human beings also recognize and appreciate me and treat me with respect and care … …

… … I trust my instincts and my feelings and I know that they protect me from getting into danger or captivity again … … and I rejoice in the freedom and honesty that I can recognize and seek in my surroundings … …

… … I accept myself and I am accepted by others … …

Behavioral Orientation and External Impact

… … I meet my fellow human beings in a friendly and open manner and at the same time allow myself to draw boundaries … … and likewise, I recognize and respect the boundaries of others who accept mine … …

… … I open myself to contact with people and step by step also approach new acquaintances … … and with every step of my openness, kind and friendly people meet me in my everyday life … …

… … I am open and at the same time allow myself to draw clear boundaries and preserve my freedom … … and my fellow human beings recognize and respect these boundaries and accept my self-determination ... ...

Success and Consolidation

... ... I am sure that by looking inward I will find myself again, and with that, I succeed more and more in standing by myself and trusting myself ... ... and I also experience acceptance and trust daily in the reactions of my fellow human beings ... ...

... ... I trust that I am strong enough to protect my freedom by drawing clear boundaries outward and communicating them ... ... and my clarity and explicitness are recognized, respected, and appreciated ... ...

... ... In my uniqueness and in my personal development, I am an enrichment for the world because I shape my life constructively and consciously ... ... and my fellow human beings are an enrichment for my own life because I can learn from them and also appreciate and accept their uniqueness ... ...

#8

Goal Formulation and Preparation

... ... You have experienced a time of violence ... ... You have found a way out, bravely left this situation, and are processing the events and occurrences of that past time ... ... Physical injuries and pain have subsided ... ... but there were and are also inner wounds ... ... Wounds of the soul ... ... Humiliation ... ... Fear ... ... Offense ... ... But you are on the path of healing ... ... both physical and emotional healing because there is great strength within you that helps you with this ... ... You have already used this inner strength and freed yourself ... ... Today you can take another big step and free yourself from the horror of the violent time ... ... from the old wounds and the feeling of powerlessness ... ... Today you find strength in yourself again ... ... Today you discover your own strength and power and can use them even more and even better to shape your life self-confidently and self-determined again ... ... to feel whole inside again ... ... A special healing begins now ... ... It begins right now ... ... Every memory is stored in our body ... ... All our potential is also stored in our body ... ... Body and soul are very closely connected ... ... And you can now use this special connection of body and soul ... ... in this trance ... ... with this hypnosis ... ...

Somato-Emotional Change

... ... Now feel your body ... ... Now, in relaxation, you feel good ... ... Your body is free of pain ... ... and your body can feel even better, become even calmer ... ... You remember the physical pain ... ... and this memory is stored in the cells of your body, but you can now think back to the time of pain and still feel good and feel a relaxed body ... ... because now everything is different ... ... The time of distress is over ... ... The time of pain is over ... ... Your body and your soul are whole again and can recover ... ... Go from head to toe along your body and concentrate on a spot where your body had a severe injury caused by violence ... ... There was more than one spot, concentrate on the first one you find ... ... on the first one that comes to your mind because it stands for all the body parts where you had bruises and injuries ... ... In every cell of your body, the memory of violence is stored, also the memory of the emotional wounds ... ... of humiliation and offense ... ... of the feeling of powerlessness and helplessness … … And at the spot you have found … … that perhaps immediately caught your eye because there was a severe injury, you can best connect with your memory … … and do the most to ensure that you can heal inside … … that the memory is only memory and the fear dissolves … … and with the fear, the offense dissolves … … and with the fear, the humiliation dissolves … … and with the fear, the uncertainty dissolves … … So concentrate on this spot of your body and feel how calm it feels today … … Imagine every breath leads there … … as if your breath flows directly to this spot of your body and heals the cells … … Maybe you wonder how that works … … how that functions … … it is very simple because also all healing and healthy memories are stored in the cells of your body … … and at special spots, you can discover and use them most easily … … Your self-healing power, your inner power to heal the body and to heal the soul, you find most easily in your heart … … So imagine that when you inhale, the air flows through your nose to your lungs and then into your heart … … With every inhalation, the air flows into your heart … … And as soon as you exhale, your self-healing power flows from your heart to the spot of the old injuries … … and heals all the wounds there ... ... When you inhale, your breath flows into the heart and when you exhale, healing energy flows into your body and your soul ... ... So breathe consciously and deliberately ... ... exactly as I have told you ... ... [Now in the breathing rhythm of the client, please!] ... ... Inhale towards the heart ... ... Exhale to old wounds ... ... Inhale and feel strength ... ... Exhale and become whole ... ... Inhale and feel strength ... ... Exhale and let go of fear ... ... Inhale and feel strength ... ... Exhale and let go of offense ... ... Inhale and feel strength ... ... Exhale and let go of fear ... ... Inhale and feel strength ... ... Exhale and let go of the past ... ... Inhale and feel strength ... ... Exhale and let go of fear ... ... Inhale and feel strength ... ... Exhale and feel healing ... ... Inhale and feel strength ... ... Exhale and feel healing ... ... good so ... ... very good so ... ...

Consolidation (Post-Hypnotic Suggestion)

... ... Continue to breathe calmly and evenly and trust that with each further breath, your body sends your own power and your own self-healing energy to all the cells ... ... Every cell of your body is informed about the healing ... ... Every cell of your body is informed that the past is only memory ... ... Every cell of your body is informed that you have built new self-confidence and build it up daily ... ... Every cell of your body is informed that you are self-confident and strong and remain self-confident and strong ... ... today and every coming day ... ...

#9

Goal Formulation and Preparation

... ... You want to find self-confidence and inner strength again ... ... You had these feelings once and today you can reactivate them ... ... that is why you are taking a special path in trance today ... ... that is why you are going on a special emotional journey in trance today ... ... It is very simple because your subconscious knows how to do it and follows my words ... ... Today you are going on a journey ... ... Today you are going on an emotional journey to a time when you were stronger than ever ... ... when you were full of self-confidence and self-assurance ... ... because these feelings are still within you ... ... They will be reactivated today ... ... maybe you wonder how you will feel it or how quickly it will happen ... ... or you just wait to see how it succeeds in being strong and self-confident again ... ...

Regression to the Time Before the Problem Arose

... ... In your feeling, you are going on a journey through space and time because this way you can find your old self-confidence again, you can reactivate your earlier strength and self-assurance … … Such a journey is very easy … … You only need to tell your subconscious which time to go to … … It should go to the time long before the violence, to a time when you felt strong and self-confident … … There was such a time … … Maybe even many years … … or only for a brief moment, the important thing is only to find this moment, to go there and reactivate the feeling of the time … … Your subconscious finds this time and goes there now, while I count from … ten … to … zero … … and when I get to zero, you are in the time when you felt strong … … stronger than ever … … ten … … nine … … eight … … seven … … six … … five … … four … … three … … two … … one … … zero … … You are strong … … You are stronger than ever … … Now … … Your self-confidence is now activated … … Your self-confidence is now available to you again … … Now … … [Approx. 20 seconds of silence] … …

Progression to the Trigger Situation

… … And now the inner journey continues and with you travels your self-confidence … … The journey now goes to the beginning of the violence, but internally you learn today to remain strong … … Your self-confidence is activated … …

Your self-confidence is fully available to you ... ... Your subconscious finds the time when your self-confidence was dissolved by and with violence ... ... You go to this point ... ... I count for you to ... ten ... and when I get to ten, you are in the time of violence and your self-confidence is with you ... ... fully and completely ... ... Your self-confidence is activated ... ... Your self-confidence is fully available to you ... ... one ... ... two ... ... three ... ... four ... ... five ... ... six ... ... seven ... ... eight ... ... nine ... ... ten ... ... You remember the violence, but you are strong ... ... You remember the violence, but you have self-confidence ... ... Your self-confidence is now activated ... ... Your self-confidence is now available to you again ... ... Now ... ... [Approx. 20 seconds of silence] ... ...

Reinterpreting the Trigger Situation

... ... If you have vivid memories, look at them because you are now in complete safety ... ... and you have your inner strength with you ... ... If you do not recognize any images, just feel deeply into your feeling because it is the feeling of that time ... ... but it felt different from fear and humiliation ... ... Today you feel strong even in the observation of the earlier time of violence ... ... and therefore you know that you can protect yourself much better from attacks now ... ... because you are strong ... ... Your self-confidence is activated and gets stronger with every breath ... ... Your subconscious helps you ... ... You can endure the memory of the violence and feel safe because your self-confidence is activated ... ... Your self-assurance is stronger than ever before ... ... and with every breath, it gets stronger ... ... You are in safety ... ... You are in complete safety ... ... and you are self-assured and strong ... ... You are truly self-assured ... ... You are truly strong ... ... [Approx. 20 seconds of silence] ... ...

Return Journey to the Present

... ... With the feeling of self-confidence, you now slowly return to the present ... ... and on the return journey, you experience something special because you bring your self-confidence fully with you ... ... Your new, activated self-assurance comes back with you and is fully available to you ... ... I count from one to ... ten ... ... and as soon as I get to ten, you are back in the present and the activated feeling of strength and self-confidence remains within you ... ... You can feel your active self-confidence as soon as you are awake again ... ... one ... ... two ... ... three ... ... four ... ... five ... ... six ... ... seven ... ... eight ... ... nine ... ... ten ... ...

You are strong ... ... You are stronger than ever ... ... Now ... ... Your self-confidence is now activated ... ... Your self-confidence is now available to you again ... ... Now and every day ... ...

#10

Arriving in the Land of Dreams

... ... There is a magical place deep in your imagination ... ... a place that only you can reach ... ... It is a place where memories linger and wait for you to look at them and learn from your own experience ... ... This place is the Land of Dreams ... ... The dreams there are like dreams at night ... ... with unexpected images and impressions that suddenly appear ... ... because feelings suddenly appear and find their way to you ... ... Maybe you know that dreams at night are visual feelings ... ... So it is in the Land of Dreams ... ... So it is in every daydream and in every fantasy ... ... So imagine being there ... ... deep in your feelings ... ... deep in your imagination ... ... deep in the Land of Dreams ... ... and wait curiously and openly for the images of the dream that show your feelings and memories ... ...

Confrontation, Clarification, and Creative Reorientation

... ... You discover a high iron fence that crosses the dreamland ... ... On your side of the fence, everything is green and alive … … On this side, you stand … … on a lush, green meadow with trees bearing ripe fruits … … There are also colorful, fresh flowers and strong shrubs here … … and small friendly animals everywhere … … You hear birds chirping and can now enjoy the beauty of life and nature on your side of the fence … … You look up and see a bright blue sky above you … … You walk to the fence … … You look to the other side … … looking through the iron bars of the fence at this gray world over there … … On the other side of the fence, everything is barren and desolate and a huge gray shadow lies on the land behind the fence … … The stormy wind on the other side blows gray sand and dust over the land where there seems to be no life … … It looks like a landscape that has long been forgotten and past … … like a land where no one lives anymore … … But on your side of the fence, everything is peaceful and beautiful … … Here, it looks like life … … Here, nature blooms and flourishes … … Here, there are plants, animals, and people … … The fence is like a border through the Land of Dreams … … a border that separates two worlds … … And through the gray sandstorm beyond the fence, a figure with a dark heavy cloak and a hood pulled over the head approaches …

... This figure comes to the fence ... ... You know this person standing there ... ... You recognize the perpetrator of the violent time ... ... You recognize the person who beat and humiliated you ... ... the once-loved person who then brought violence into your life ... ... Motionless, he stands on his side of the fence ... ... Here in the Land of Dreams, only you decide what is possible ... ... No one who is not invited by you can cross the fence and be with you in the Land of Dreams ... ... not even him ... ... This person is not here for his own sake ... ... It does not matter what motives he once had or what his story was ... ... Like you, he also has a Land of his Dreams, as we all do, there he can find his story if he is ready for it ... ... Here it is only about you and your peace ... ... only for that reason is he here today ... ... only for that reason ... ... You consider what you want to say to him ... ... You may tell him about the feelings and fear you once had ... ... when violence was still the order of the day ... ... Tell him also the feelings that perhaps only you know, which you have never spoken to anyone about but perhaps can now feel as a memory ... ... Take your time to tell this person about it ... ... If you want, tell him about it, if you want, shout it at him ... ... Do it as your feeling tells you because now you have to fulfill nothing, keep no composure, and play no role, because that would be a renewed demand in your life to behave differently than your true feeling ... ... Such demands were too often ... ... In the Land of Dreams, there are no demands ... ... You are not here to forgive but to free yourself ... ... Say now in the Land of Dreams what you want or must say ... ... I am with you and give you some time ... ... [Now make a felt minute pause and let the client go into inner contact to feel and speak their feelings internally.] ... ... You are still standing at the fence between the worlds and the person on the other side turns into a stone sculpture ... ... He can no longer move, can do nothing to you, can do nothing at all because the time of then is long past ... ... The world on the other side of the fence is a shadow of the past ... ... Whatever the perpetrator of then could do today, the done cannot be changed ... ... It is part of your story ... ... The part of this person on the shadow side that you once loved because he was without violence and horror, that part lives somewhere in the Land of your Dreams, as a memory ... ... But the part of violence that frightened you, that was so terrible and bad, stands as a stone sculpture beyond the fence and crumbles to dust that is blown away by the wind ... ...

Mindfulness and Self-Loyalty

... ... And you turn around and walk step by step, deeper and deeper, into the blooming land on your side of the fence ... ... On your way, you think about the fact that you can be free forever because the Land of Dreams always and anytime helps you to be free and stay free ... ... But where is this Land of Dreams? ... ... Is it real? ... ... Yes, it is real ... ... The Land of Dreams lies deep within you and has always been there ... ... I am just telling you about it ... ...

Distribution, publication, and copying in any form are prohibited and subject to damages.

Overview of All Titles in the Series "Ten Hypnoses"

Volume 1: Smoking Cessation
Volume 2: Anxiety and Restlessness
Volume 3: Burnout
Volume 4: Reducing Overweight
Volume 5: Coping with the Past
Volume 6: Suicidal Thoughts and Attempts
Volume 7: Psycho-Oncology
Volume 8: Obsessions and Tics
Volume 9: Self-Confidence and Decision-Making
Volume 10: Grief Work
Volume 11: Psychosomatics
Volume 12: Chronic Pain
Volume 13: Depressive Thoughts
Volume 14: Panic Attacks
Volume 15: Domestic Violence, Victim Support
Volume 16: Post-Traumatic Stress
Volume 17: Exam Anxiety and Stage Fright
Volume 18: Anti-Violence Training, Offender Support
Volume 19: Addiction Tendencies
Volume 20: Social Phobia and Fear of Contact
Volume 21: Nail Biting
Volume 22: Self-Awareness and Self-Love
Volume 23: Teeth Grinding and Night Clenching
Volume 24: Feelings of Guilt
Volume 25: Fear in Crowds
Volume 26: Fear of Flying, Aviophobia
Volume 27: Fear in Enclosed Spaces, Claustrophobia
Volume 28: Tinnitus, Ear Noises
Volume 29: Fear of Heights
Volume 30: Neurodermatitis

Copying, publishing, and sharing with third parties are only permitted with the written consent of the author. Please observe the notes on copyright and usage.

Volume 31: Finding Inner Balance
Volume 32: Overcoming Loneliness
Volume 33: Fear of Illness, Hypochondria
Volume 34: Anticipatory Anxiety, Fear of Fear
Volume 35: Jealousy in Relationships
Volume 36: Driving Anxiety
Volume 37: New Start after Separation
Volume 38: Fear of Injections
Volume 39: Heart Anxiety Neurosis
Volume 40: Overcoming Resentment and Anger
Volume 41: Resolving Blockages and Positive Thinking
Volume 42: Stress Reduction, Stress Management
Volume 43: Body Relaxation
Volume 44: Deep Relaxation
Volume 45: Fear of the Dark
Volume 46: Falling Asleep and Staying Asleep
Volume 47: Compulsive Buying
Volume 48: Restless Legs Syndrome
Volume 49: Bulimia
Volume 50: Anorexia
Volume 51: Overcoming Nightmares
Volume 52: Imagined Deformity
Volume 53: Overcoming Distrust, Finding Trust
Volume 54: Processing Failures
Volume 55: Humiliation, Emotional Hurt
Volume 56: Distressing Compassion, Vicarious Suffering
Volume 57: Self-Forgiveness
Volume 58: Self-Awareness, Self-Confidence
Volume 59: Saying No
Volume 60: Assertiveness
Volume 61: Setting Boundaries and Self-Assertion
Volume 62: Decision-Making Ability

Volume 63: Success Orientation
Volume 64: Ruminating, Circular Thinking
Volume 65: Accepting Pregnancy
Volume 66: Birth Preparation
Volume 67: Spiritual Opening
Volume 68: Joy of Life and Inner Lightness
Volume 69: Patience and Inner Peace
Volume 70: Fibromyalgia and Rheumatism
Volume 71: Irritable Bowel Syndrome, Crohn's Disease
Volume 72: Fear of Nausea, Emetophobia
Volume 73: Stuttering and Cluttering, Speech Flow Disorders
Volume 74: Concentration and Knowledge Anchoring
Volume 75: Vitality and Spontaneity
Volume 76: Searching for Meaning and Finding Goals
Volume 77: Life Crises, Life Events
Volume 78: Workaholism, Goal Obsession
Volume 79: Helper Syndrome, Helpless Helpers
Volume 80: Medication Abuse
Volume 81: Gambling Addiction
Volume 82: Internet Addiction, Smartphone Addiction
Volume 83: Hoarding Disorder, Compulsive Collecting
Volume 84: Conspiracy Thoughts, Overvalued Ideas
Volume 85: Fear of Operations and Treatments
Volume 86: Fear of Aging
Volume 87: Travel Anxiety
Volume 88: Anxiety When Urinating, Paruresis
Volume 89: Fear of Intimacy and Togetherness
Volume 90: Fear of Blushing
Volume 91: Coming Out in Homosexuality
Volume 92: Charisma Training
Volume 93: Migraines and Chronic Headaches
Volume 94: Overcoming Allergies, Bronchial Asthma

Volume 95: Normalizing Blood Pressure
Volume 96: Compulsive Perfectionism
Volume 97: Sports Hypnosis, Motivation
Volume 98: Sports Hypnosis, Performance Enhancement
Volume 99: Determination and Focus
Volume 100: Encountering the Inner Child
Volume 101: Cravings, Binge Eating
Volume 102: Stimulating Metabolism
Volume 103: Bipolar Mood Swings
Volume 104: Borderline, Identity Crises
Volume 105: Hypomania, Euphoria, Mania
Volume 106: Restlessness, Agitation
Volume 107: Nervous Breakdown
Volume 108: Adjustment Disorders
Volume 109: Self-Alienation, Depersonalization
Volume 110: Ending Self-Pity
Volume 111: Primary Gain of Illness
Volume 112: Secondary Gain of Illness
Volume 113: Bullying, Victim Support
Volume 114: Letting Go of Envy and Jealousy
Volume 115: Fear of Spiders, Arachnophobia
Volume 116: Fear of Dogs or Cats
Volume 117: Fear of Strangers, Xenophobia
Volume 118: Excessive Worries, Generalized Anxiety
Volume 119: Strengthening Sense of Responsibility
Volume 120: Unrequited Love, Heartache
Volume 121: Work-Life Balance
Volume 122: Letting Go of Unattainable Goals
Volume 123: Allowing and Accepting Help
Volume 124: Letting Go of Adult Children
Volume 125: Tourette Syndrome
Volume 126: Life Changes and New Starts

Volume 127: Accepting Life in a Wheelchair
Volume 128: Understanding and Overcoming Homesickness
Volume 129: Understanding and Overcoming Wanderlust
Volume 130: Dizziness, Meniere's Disease
Volume 131: Overcoming Aggression
Volume 132: Cutting and Self-Harm
Volume 133: Hair Pulling, Trichotillomania
Volume 134: Postpartum Depression
Volume 135: For Relatives of Dementia Patients
Volume 136: Self-Harm, Artificial Disorders
Volume 137: Activating Self-Healing Powers
Volume 138: Preventing Depression Relapse
Volume 139: Reactive Psychoses, Follow-Up
Volume 140: Obsessive Thoughts and Impulses
Volume 141: Compulsive Checking
Volume 142: Compulsive Counting, Symmetry Obsession
Volume 143: Compulsive Washing, Cleanliness Obsession
Volume 144: Compulsive Questioning
Volume 145: Dissociative Paralysis
Volume 146: Phantom Pain
Volume 147: Overcoming Complaining
Volume 148: Hay Fever, Pollen Allergy
Volume 149: Sexual Abuse, Victim Support
Volume 150: Standing Strong Against Sexism, #metoo
Volume 151: Binge Eating
Volume 152: Overcoming Thoughts of Revenge
Volume 153: Detachment from the Aggressor, Stockholm Syndrome
Volume 154: Courage to Separate
Volume 155: Chronic Fatigue, Exhaustion
Volume 156: Fear of the Future, Existential Anxiety
Volume 157: Excessive Worry About Children
Volume 158: Fear of Failure

Volume 159: Ending Distrust and Control
Volume 160: Dejection, Dysphoria
Volume 161: Boreout, Chronic Boredom
Volume 162: Bipolar Disorders, Relapse Prevention
Volume 163: Mania, Relapse Prevention
Volume 164: Nihilism, Feelings of Worthlessness
Volume 165: Thumb Sucking
Volume 166: Being Brave
Volume 167: Being Proud
Volume 168: Overcoming Shyness
Volume 169: Being Able to Delegate Responsibility
Volume 170: Being Able to Show Emotions
Volume 171: Letting Go of Guilt, Victim Support
Volume 172: Processing Guilt, Offender Support
Volume 173: Mood Swings, Cyclothymia
Volume 174: Lack of Drive, Vital Sadness
Volume 175: Hearing Voices with Reality Reference
Volume 176: Confident Communication
Volume 177: Standing Up for Oneself
Volume 178: Taking New Paths
Volume 179: Confident Job Application
Volume 180: No Longer Being Taken Advantage Of
Volume 181: End of Submissiveness
Volume 182: Depressive Numbness
Volume 183: Mood Drops, Affective Incontinence
Volume 184: Mood Instability
Volume 185: Somatoform Disorders
Volume 186: Stomach Ulcer, Psychosomatic
Volume 187: Accepting Amputation
Volume 188: Overcoming and Letting Go of Hatred
Volume 189: Ending Accusations
Volume 190: Allowing Tears, Being Able to Cry

Volume 191: Finding and Sorting Repressed Feelings
Volume 192: Somatoform Pain
Volume 193: Living Autonomously
Volume 194: Anhedonia, Joylessness
Volume 195: Persistent Sadness
Volume 196: Obesity, Food Addiction
Volume 197: Parents of Abused Children
Volume 198: Letting Go and Letting Be
Volume 199: Childhood Sexual Abuse
Volume 200: Fear of Loss

www.ingramcontent.com/pod-product-compliance
Lightning Source LLC
Chambersburg PA
CBHW030502220526
45464CB00006B/2627